Lemon Fresh

A Beginner's Guide to Unlocking the Power of Lemongrass Oil

By
Clarice M. Pines

<u>DISCLAIMER</u>

Content

Introduction

Lemongrass oil, originating from Southeast Asia, has been an integral part of traditional medicine and local customs for centuries. Its use dates back thousands of years in traditional Indian medicine, where it was used to treat infectious illnesses and fever. The Chinese used it to treat a variety of conditions such as colds, rheumatism, and infectious diseases. Additionally, lemongrass was utilized in spiritual cleansing rituals to protect, purify and promote peace. Apart from its medicinal properties, lemongrass is widely used as an ingredient in various cuisines, including Thai, Caribbean, Vietnamese, and South Asian. Its citrus aroma and lemony flavor make it an excellent choice for adding exotic flavors to recipes.

Lemongrass oil is also frequently used for flavoring soups and teas, and as a fragrant addition to soaps, shampoos, cosmetics, and homemade deodorizers. With the recent surge of interest in essential oils worldwide and their growing popularity in the United States, Lemongrass essential oil has emerged as one of the most highly sought-after oils in aromatherapy today. The reasons behind its popularity are clear. With its potent medicinal and therapeutic properties, lemongrass oil is used topically to alleviate muscle pain, repel insects, and combat bacterial infections. Additionally, it can be consumed internally to aid in digestion. This oil possesses strong anti-inflammatory, antibacterial, antiviral, antifungal, and antiseptic properties, making it a highly effective remedy for various health issues. Its broad range of benefits has made it a go-to solution for many who seek natural healing and wellness.

In this book, you will discover that lemongrass essential oil has the potential to alleviate several medical conditions. It should be noted, however, that lemongrass oil is not a substitute for professional medical care. Nevertheless, scientific research is starting to support the traditional uses and benefits of this oil, making it a valuable addition to many healthcare routines, with the approval and close monitoring of a doctor, especially in the case of internal use. The book provides a comprehensive list of the many benefits and uses of lemongrass essential oil. While generally safe to use, there are instances where lemongrass oil may cause skin irritation or have harmful effects if ingested incorrectly. Therefore, the book will also discuss necessary precautions that must be taken to ensure the safe and appropriate use of the oil.

Lemon Grass and Its Benefits

Lemongrass oil is a highly beneficial substance that provides numerous health advantages. It possesses astringent, analgesic, antipyretic, antidepressant, antimicrobial, antiseptic, anti-inflammatory, diuretic, bactericidal, deodorant, galactagogue, sedative, nervine, febrifuge, tonic, fungicidal and carminative properties. Obtained through steam distillation of the leaves of the lemongrass plant, also known as Andropogon Citratus and Cymbopogon Citratus, its main constituents include citral, geranyl acetate, limonene, myrcene, farnesol, nerol, neral, citronellal, geraniol, terpineol, , methyl and heptenone. Despite its name, the scent of lemongrass is sweeter, milder and less sour than that of lemons. As a fast-growing plant that provides a wide range of health benefits, lemongrass oil has become a popular commodity in both mainstream and organic markets.

Before we explore the extensive benefits of lemongrass oil, let's first understand what makes this essential oil so unique based on scientific evidence and research gathered over the years. In 2012, a study was conducted to evaluate the antibacterial properties of lemongrass. The researchers used a disk diffusion method to test the effect of lemongrass essential oil on Staphylococcal, a bacterium that causes a group of infections called staph infections. The results showed that lemongrass oil effectively disrupted the infection, proving its antibacterial properties. Another study tested the antifungal effects of lemongrass essential oil on Candida, a type of fungal infection that can affect various parts of the body. The researchers used disk diffusion tests to examine the antifungal properties of lemongrass oil, and the results demonstrated that it has the ability to reduce the effects of Candida.

In 2009, a study was conducted to determine the effectiveness of geranium and lemongrass essential oil vapors in reducing airborne and surface-level bacteria. The study produced varied results based on the methods used. In an office setting, the presence of airborne bacteria decreased by 89% within 15 hours, while the growth of bacteria on seeded plates in a sealed box was reduced by 35% within 20 hours. This study confirms that lemongrass essential oil can be used for air disinfection. With this scientific evidence in mind, let's now move on to discussing the numerous benefits of lemongrass essential oil. These benefits include:

Astringent

An astringent is a chemical substance that prevents blood discharge by contracting bodily tissues. When a person is bleeding heavily, an astringent is used to accelerate the clotting process (Hemostasis) and stop the flow of blood in order to preserve their life. Lemongrass, with its astringent characteristics, aids in a variety of ways. It not only stops bleeding and helps healing, but it also prevents the loosening and falling of your teeth and hair by encouraging the contraction of gums and hair follicles.

Analgesic

Medicines containing analgesic, a pain reliever, can help decrease inflammation and discomfort. Lemongrass essential oil appears to have analgesic qualities due to the presence of a chemical component known as myrcene. It can successfully relieve joint and muscular pain, as well as headaches and toothaches caused by viral illnesses such as a cold, influenza, or fever. Also, if you suffer from general body discomfort as a result of athletics and physical activities, this essential oil might be beneficial.

Antipyretic

An antipyretic is a substance, such as a medicine or plant, that helps to reduce your body's temperature, resulting in a reduction in fever. Since this is comparable to a febrifuge, it is also beneficial in lowering excessive fever. As a result, if you have a high fever, lemongrass essential oil can be used to keep it from reaching harmful levels. Lemongrass is well-known and used for its antipyretic effects, and it is frequently provided in tea for the same reason.

Antidepressant

Lemongrass is good for stress-related illnesses since it contains antidepressant effects. Lemongrass essential oil may enhance confidence, improve mental strength, elevate spirits, and keep depression at bay if you want to feel calm, rejuvenated, and regenerated. This may be particularly beneficial in driving away depression caused by a loss in the family or failure in your work. In fact, lemongrass might help you relax and ease anxiety. Lemongrass essential oil can help those suffering from ailments such as panic attacks, anxiety disorders, and depression.

Antimicrobial

Lemongrass oil, because of its powerful antibacterial characteristics, inhibits bacterial and microbial development in the body, both outwardly and inside! It has also been demonstrated to suppress bacterial infections in the urinary tract, stomach, colon, respiratory system, and other organs. Not only that, but lemongrass essential oil can help heal ailments caused by microbial or bacterial infections, such as malaria, typhoid, and food poisoning

Antiseptic

Lemongrass essential oil has antibacterial characteristics, making it ideal for treating interior and exterior wounds. This is why essential oils are commonly used in antimicrobial creams and lotions. If you cut yourself, using lemongrass essential oil to the wound can keep it from becoming infected and keep it from becoming septic.

Anti-Inflammatory

Most people experience extreme discomfort and suffering as a result of chronic inflammation, making it difficult to carry out daily tasks. Yet, because lemongrass has anti-inflammatory characteristics, its oil can help relieve discomfort caused by inflammation, such as in your back or muscles. Also, if you suffer from stomach cramps and farts on a regular basis, lemongrass essential oil might bring much-needed relief.

Diuretic

The usage of lemongrass essential oil increases both the quantity and frequency of urine. You may dismiss this as inconsequential, yet frequent urinating is really advantageous to your health. When a person urinates, 4% of the urine volume is made up of fat, which is removed from the body. As a result, the more you urinate, the more fat you will lose. Urination aids digestion and helps to avoid gas production. It helps to minimize edema and eliminate extra water from the body. The most essential benefit, however, is its capacity to lower blood pressure. That is why, in order to reduce blood pressure, most pharmacological treatments and pharmaceuticals cause frequent urine. Urination also helps to cleanse the kidneys and eliminate toxins from the body.

Deodorant

Lemongrass has a pleasant and delicate citrus aroma, which is why the plant is grown for its fragrance as well. Lemongrass essential oil is a great natural alternative to synthetic deodorants on the market today. They are not only costly, but they also have a long-term environmental impact. Moreover, these deodorants can occasionally aggravate allergies and cause skin irritation. Lemongrass essential oil, on the other hand, is a natural substance that performs none of the aforementioned things. In fact, in diluted form, it functions as an excellent deodorant with no negative effects. Additionally, because it is non-toxic to the person or the environment, more people are turning to lemongrass oil as a natural air freshener or deodorizer.

Fungicidal

Lemongrass essential oil possesses fungicidal effects, according to study. As a result, if you have fungal illnesses such as ringworm or athlete's foot, lemongrass essential oil can be used to cure them.

Febrifuge

Lemongrass essential oil's febrifuge qualities aid to reduce fever while fighting the diseases that cause it. It also stimulates perspiration, which causes toxins to be sweated out.

Galactagogue

A galactogogue is any chemical or agent that stimulates milk production in the breasts. It is also thought to boost milk quality. This is especially beneficial for nursing women who must feed their infants. Although lemongrass essential oil's galactagogue qualities promote milk supply, it also helps newborns prevent infections. As you are surely aware, babies are more susceptible to illnesses. Yet, the antibacterial and antimicrobial qualities of lemongrass essential oil come into action and are absorbed in the milk, safeguarding the infant from developing infections.

Insecticidal

Lemongrass has been used to repel insects for ages due to its excellent insecticidal capabilities. Even now, it's a well-known and extensively used insect repellent. It successfully destroys insects while also keeping them at bay. But, there isn't enough study available right now to know exactly which insects it can affect. Thus we can't truly guarantee that it will get rid of cockroaches.

Nervine

According to most medical professionals, lemongrass is a nerve that functions as a general tonic for the nervous system. It can aid in the treatment of a variety of nerve illnesses, including lack of reflexes, trembling hands (or limbs), sluggishness, anxiousness, convulsions, vertigo, Parkinson's disease, and Alzheimer's disease. As a result, utilizing lemongrass essential oil can help to strengthen and invigorate the nerves throughout your body.

Sedative

One of the most valued and vital medical characteristics of lemongrass essential oil is its ability to act as a relaxing and sedative in nature. Lemongrass essential oil lowers anxiety, heals inflammation, and soothes skin irritation due to its relaxing, soothing, and sedating effects on the psyche.

Tonic

Lemongrass essential oil is also a tonic (a chemical or agent that improves health) for the mind and body. It tones all of your body's systems, from the digestive and respiratory systems to the excretory and neurological systems. Not only that, but it also improves nutrition absorption in the body, strengthening the immune system and giving much-needed strength.

Negative Side Effects

Lemongrass essential oil is typically safe for most individuals to use, whether in food, on the skin, or orally. Lemongrass oil, on the other hand, may create redness or a burning feeling if you have sensitive skin. As a result, it is advised that you start with tiny amounts or combine the lemongrass essential oil with a quality carrier oil to ensure that it does not irritate your skin. Furthermore, because lemongrass essential oil promotes menstrual flow, pregnant women should avoid using it at least until the birth of their child, as there is a tiny risk of miscarriage.

While lemongrass essential oil is a Galactogogue, certain medical professionals do not suggest it for nursing moms. The same holds true for utilizing lemongrass essential oil on youngsters.

Lemongrass Oil's Many Applications

Although lemongrass oil has been around for generations, its application is now more important than ever. Lemongrass oil is becoming increasingly popular due to its numerous health and wellness advantages. The oil not only smells great, but it also cures your body and brain on a molecular level. Since lemongrass oil may be utilized effectively in healing and supporting your mental and physical well-being, let's look at how you can benefit from this wonderful essential oil:

Muscle Relaxer

Lemongrass oil, with its potent anti-inflammatory effects, aids in the improvement of blood circulation throughout the body, successfully relieving cramps, sprains, backaches, and muscular spasms. This formula is great for temporary pain relief. Just combine 2 drops of lemongrass oil with a carrier oil (jojoba oil works best) and apply on your skin.

Pain Relieving

Lemongrass oil offers relaxing and therapeutic effects that can help ease headache discomfort, stress, or pressure. The oil is thought to relieve allergy-related headaches and is especially beneficial for people who are allergic to peppermint, which is typically advised as an essential oil for headache relief. Headaches are best relieved physically, so mix 2 drops of lemongrass oil with 1 teaspoon of carrier oil, such as jojoba oil, and massage over broad regions of your head. You should feel better right away.

Menstrual Cramp Treatment

While lemongrass oil is known to promote menstrual flow, which is why pregnant women should avoid using it, lemongrass tea can aid women suffering from monthly cramps. Indeed, it can assist with the associated nausea and irritation. Drink two cups of lemongrass tea every day to help alleviate period discomfort. The tea is widely accessible in most health food and grocery stores.

Wound Healing

A few drops of lemongrass oil combined with a saline solution can help clean and wash out wounds. Afterwards, mix the oil with some Salve for an antiseptic treatment and cover the wounds with gauze or bandage to keep dirt out.

Sleep Aid and Stress Reducer

Lemongrass oil's pleasant and relaxing smell is believed to alleviate sleeplessness, irritation, and anxiety. Not to add, the oil's hypnotic and sedative effects can aid increase sleep quality and duration. Add 5 to 6 drops of lemongrass oil to your diffuser or place a drop on your palm and inhale deeply to ease tension and enhance sleep.

Augmentation of Mood

Lemongrass oil's earthy and fresh aroma makes it ideal for use in a diffuser. It improves confidence, mental wellness, and helps keep depression at bay. Use 5 drops of lemongrass oil in your diffuser to feel rested, rejuvenated, and regenerated. Massage 3 drops of diluted lemongrass oil across your chest and hop into a hot shower or bath for a more immediate benefit.

Then, as you breathe in the oil particles, exhale to relieve stress and raise your mood.

Treatment of Shock

Whenever someone is in shock, whether as a result of an accident or a medical condition (such as heatstroke, allergies, or poisoning), quick care is required to minimize the consequences. And lemongrass oil can be really beneficial in this aspect. Just sprinkle 2 drops of the oil on a cotton ball and place it under the victim's nostrils to comfort and quiet them until aid comes.

Enhancer of Energy

If you've run out of energy and are feeling fatigued and sluggish, lemongrass oil can help. To give yourself a natural energy boost before your training sessions, combine 3-4 drops of lemongrass, peppermint, and wild orange essential oils in your diffuser.

Skin Care

One significant advantage of lemongrass oil is its skin healing abilities. As a result, lemongrass is frequently used in lotions, soaps, shampoos, oils, and conditioners.

It cleanses all skin types well, and its astringent and antibacterial characteristics provide even and luminous skin by sterilizing your pores, strengthening your skin tissues, and acting as a natural toner. Add one drop of lemongrass oil to a carrier oil and apply to affected areas once or twice a day to clear up acne. Add one drop of lemongrass oil to warm water and use as a skin rinse for oily skin.

Natural Deodorant

Lemongrass essential oil is a natural and healthy deodorizer and air freshener. All you have to do is use an oil diffuser/vaporizer or mix a few drops of this fragrant oil with water to make a mist. Other essential oils, such as peppermint or lavender, can be used to create a bespoke aroma.

Natural Insect Repellent

Lemongrass oil is extensively used to repel insects such as ants and mosquitoes because of its high geraniol and citral content. Because of its moderate aroma, this natural insect repellent may be applied directly on your skin. In fact, the oil may be used to kill fleas as well. You may apply the spray to your pet's coat after adding 5 drops of lemongrass essential oil to water.

Hair Care

If you suffer from hair loss or an irritated and itchy scalp, you'll be relieved to hear that lemongrass oil may heal greasy hair, battle hair loss, and cure scalp issues. It is also thought to strengthen hair follicles, which is necessary to prevent hair loss. To cure hair, lemongrass oil is frequently blended with lavender and rosemary oil. Just combine 1 tablespoon of jojoba or another carrier oil with 3-4 drops of lemongrass essential oil and let it on your hair for 15-30 minutes. Next, as usual, wash your hair.

Detoxifying

Because of its diuretic qualities, lemongrass oil is utilized as a detoxifier in many nations throughout the world. It is well-known for cleansing the pancreas, digestive tract, bladder, kidneys, and liver. Combine a few drops of lemongrass oil with grapefruit or ginger essential oil and add it to your tea or soup to eliminate harmful toxins from your body and maintain your system clean.

Antioxidant Properties

Lemongrass oil, according to research, has the power to prevent free radicals from significantly harming one's health. One of its key components, citral, is known to suppress cancer cell proliferation early on. Yet, the oil's anti-cancer properties are particularly prominent in the prevention of skin cancer. If you have cancer and are receiving chemotherapy or radiation treatments, adding a few drops of lemongrass oil to your tea will improve the healing process.

Fights Flu and Colds

Lemongrass oil has antibacterial qualities that can help fight germs and cure illnesses like the common cold. It is also known to have a cooling effect, which aids in the reduction of body temperature when you have a fever. To kill flu and flu viruses, combine a few drops of lemongrass oil with a carrier oil (jojoba or coconut oil) and apply it around your ears and up your throat. You should instantly feel relieved.

Reducer of Inflammation

Lemongrass oil contains limonene, which has powerful anti-inflammatory effects. According to research, inflammation is linked to practically every medical condition and is crucial in allergic illnesses such as arthritis, diabetes, high cholesterol, and cardiovascular disease, among others. This dish will naturally assist to decrease inflammation in the body. Just combine 2-3 drops of lemongrass oil with a carrier oil and apply straight to the inflammatory area of the body.

Precautions You Must Take

For all the right reasons, lemongrass oil is becoming increasingly popular in aromatherapy mixes and natural health treatments. Yet, because it is a very concentrated liquid, it can be harmful if not utilized correctly. This does not exclude you from utilizing lemongrass essential oil (or any other essential oil for that matter). Although there is continuous debate over the safety of essential oils, the reality is that when used appropriately, they are amazing natural treatments. The same is true with Lemongrass oil. We are not attempting to frighten you away from using it, but rather to encourage you to conduct adequate research and, more importantly, to take safeguards.

The suggestions below are meant to assist make the usage of lemongrass essential oil safe for you and others around you. If you have any reservations or specific queries about your medical situation, you should visit your doctor immediately. A skilled aromatherapy practitioner can also provide instruction and advice.

1. Keep lemongrass oil out of the reach of youngsters at all times. To avoid the potential of accidental consumption, all essential oils should be treated like over-the-counter drugs or antibiotics.

Absolutely, if babies and children consume lemongrass oil, they can become deadly.

2. Never apply undiluted lemongrass oil to your skin since it may create an allergic response or skin irritation. Always dilute your oil with suitable carrier oils before application.

3. When using lemongrass oil (either as an individual oil or in a mix of oils), never use more than the amount needed to complete the task. For example, if you only need two drops, use two rather than three or four.

4. It is usually a good idea to properly wash your hands after handling undiluted/pure lemongrass oil. While you may not be allergic to the oil, someone else most likely is. There is no solid evidence that enough essential oils may permeate the skin to produce systemic toxicity, but it's best to be cautious than sorry.

5. Use only pure, therapeutic-grade lemongrass oil and follow the instructions and warnings on the packaging.

6. If you are new to essential oils and aromatherapy, a skin patch test is recommended to discover chemical sensitivities. Lemongrass oil, like other essential oils, can cause allergic responses or sensitization in sensitive people. Place one small drop of diluted lemongrass oil on the inside of your elbow to do a skin patch test. Avoid using the oil if you notice discomfort, irritation, or redness within 24 hours. Remember that washing with water will not help. Instead, massage the afflicted region with vegetable oil (such as olive oil).

7. Avoid getting lemongrass oil in your eyes. If it gets into your eyes, dilute it with vegetable oil rather than water.

8. Pregnant women should see their physician before taking lemongrass oil or any other essential oil. As previously stated, because lemongrass oil promotes menstrual flow, it may cause preterm contractions or miscarriage.

9. If you have a medical problem, such as epilepsy, hypertension, asthma, or liver damage, see your doctor before taking lemongrass oil since it may conflict with your prescription drugs.

10. Because not all essential oils are made equal, always purchase lemongrass oil from recognised essential oil vendors.

Lemongrass Oil and Photosensitivity

Lemongrass can induce photosensitivity, hence it should not be applied to the skin before being exposed to UV rays or sunlight. Chemical ingredients may degrade, resulting in skin discoloration, rashes, or even burns. As a result, it is strongly suggested that you avoid the sun after applying lemongrass oil. Be especially cautious if you have applied the oil to your feet or regions beneath your clothing.

Lemongrass Oil Storage

When citrus oils, such as lemongrass oil, are exposed to sunshine and air, they deteriorate quickly. As a result, the oil's medicinal effects may deteriorate with time. After a time, you may notice a significant shift in the scent of your lemongrass oil.

Store the oil in amber glass bottles or jars to prevent degradation. Wondering \why? This is due to the fact that dark tinted glass, such as amber, filters solar rays, which may hasten degradation. Moreover, ensure that the bottles or jars containing the oil are securely sealed and stored in a dark, cold area.

Lemongrass Oil Toxicity

Lemongrass oil is made up of several ingredients. Some elements may be hazardous to susceptible people, especially infants, newborns, pregnant and elderly women. Toxicity can occur from either oral intake or improper application or inhalation of the oil. As a result, it is suggested that you observe the label's directions and cautions.

Another thing to keep in mind is that essential oils are extremely concentrated goods. Even non-toxic oils can be quite poisonous if used in large quantities. One drop of lemongrass oil, or any other essential oil, is approximately comparable to 20-35 g of the plant itself. Hence, utilizing the correct balance is critical to avoiding the hazardous effects of lemongrass oil.

Conclusion

Lemongrass essential oil, as you can see, may be utilized for a variety of health-related applications. The multiple benefits of this remarkable essential oil may be employed by almost everyone, from lowering inflammation and stress to inhibiting the growth of inflammation and even cancer. But, as previously said, in order to get the advantages of lemongrass oil, it is critical to utilize the essential oil correctly and safely. Thus, obey the instructions and cautions on the label, store your oil appropriately, and prioritize safety. This manner, you will be able to reap its benefits without any difficulty.

* 9 7 9 8 3 9 0 0 0 1 6 6 0 *